BREAK FREE!
RECLAIM YOUR POWER

Practical guides for a healthy relationship with your adult child

Jessica Rodriquez

Table of content

Chapter one
Chapter two
Chapter three
Chapter four
Chapter five
Chapter six

Chapter one

<u>**Reflect and Assess**</u>

It's time to consider your current relationships with your adult children. Examine the situations where you feel your authority is being undermined or your boundaries are being crossed. Determine the particular actions or circumstances that need to change.

Locate a Quiet Area: Find a place that is quiet and comfortable where you can reflect without interruptions, and set aside a specific time for it. It could be a quiet area of your home, a park, or any other setting that makes you feel at ease.

Self-Reflection: Consider your feelings, ideas, and experiences in relation to your relationship with your adult child as a starting point. Consider the following inquiries for yourself:

- What do I think of the dynamics with my adult child right now?
- What specific actions or behaviors from my adult child cause me to feel as though my authority has been diminished?
- How do these dynamics affect my general happiness and well-being?

- Are there any recurring patterns or circumstances that require modification?
- What are my personal wants and needs in this relationship?

Give yourself permission to be honest and open with your thoughts and feelings. To clarify your thoughts, jot them down in a journal or notebook.

Establish Boundaries: Think about the areas with your adult child where you need to set boundaries. Think about the following elements:

Emotional Boundaries:

- Are there any particular subjects or exchanges that always make you feel drained or overburdened?

- Are you entangled in your adult child's emotional problems all the time?

- Do you feel as though your personal time and space are being violated or disrespected?

- Are your adult child's expectations stressing you out or taking up too much of your time?

- Financial restrictions: Does your adult child have any demands or expectations that you find to be unjustified or unsustainable?

Personal Autonomy: Does your adult child's behavior interfere with your right to make independent decisions?

Make clear and precise notes of the boundaries you want to impose in each area.

Analyze the patterns of communication: Consider the ways in which you and your adult child communicate. Think about the following:

When you voice your ideas and concerns, do you feel heard and respected?

Do your conversations frequently involve manipulation or guilt-tripping? Are you frequently ignored or interrupted?

Do you feel confident invoking your needs and establishing boundaries in conversation?

Consider how your sense of control and power within the relationship is affected by these communication styles.

Analyze the Impact: Consider how your overall wellbeing, happiness, and other relationships are affected by the current dynamics with your adult child. Think about it.

Are there any unfavorable physical or emotional effects of the present circumstances?

What impact does it have on your marriage, your relationships with your family members, and your close friendships?

Has your adult child's influence caused you to postpone or neglect any aspects of your life?

You'll be able to appreciate the importance of reclaiming your power when you are aware of the bigger picture.

Think About Outside Perspectives: Ask for advice from therapists, family members, or trusted friends who can offer an objective viewpoint. Ask for their observations and insights as you share your reflections with them. Others may occasionally be able to help you see patterns you may have missed or provide insightful commentary.

Study Child Development: Think about how your child's upbringing might have impacted the current dynamics. Think about it:

- Did their upbringing establish any patterns that are part of the current power structure?
- Have you ever failed to set appropriate boundaries or unintentionally encourage certain behaviors?

Think about your own parenting approach and how it might have influenced the dynamics of your relationships. Knowing the origins of the dynamic can help you understand how it has developed and guide your strategy for regaining power.

Find Patterns and Triggers: Make a note of any patterns or triggers that recur frequently in your interactions with your adult child. This might include particular actions, circumstances, or subjects that frequently cause conflict or produce power disparities. Understanding these triggers will improve your ability to anticipate and avoid them.

Consider asking for feedback from a therapist or counselor who can offer unbiased perceptions of the dynamics between you and your adult child. They can assist you in gaining more clarity and recognizing any blind spots or underlying problems that contribute to the power disparity. Assess Your Emotional Reactions: Be aware of your feelings as you interact with your adult child. Keep an eye out for any frustration, rage, guilt, or fear that might appear. This awareness can assist you in realizing how your emotions might be affecting your capacity to assert your authority and establish boundaries.

Take stock of your personal development and self-awareness as you reflect on them:Think about any alterations or advancements in other spheres of your life.Your confidence will be boosted, and you'll be reminded of your ability to improve the parent-child relationship by thinking back on your own development.

Think About the Long-Term Gains: Think about the long-term advantages of taking back your power and establishing sound boundaries. This might entail fostering a more harmonious and respectful relationship, encouraging personal development and independence for both you and your adult child, and establishing a more favorable family environment.

You can develop a deeper understanding of your emotions, needs, and the specific areas where you need to reclaim power from your adult child by engaging in a thorough reflection and assessment process. This self-awareness will lay the groundwork for setting healthy boundaries and promoting a more reasonable and harmonious relationship.

Always keep in mind that reflection and assessment are ongoing processes. Continue to assess and modify your strategy as you proceed through the process of reclaiming power in light of your developing insights and experiences. As you work to develop a healthier and more satisfying relationship with your adult child, have patience with both of you.

Chapter two

<u>Define your boundaries</u>

Your personal boundaries, values, and expectations should be made very clear. Decide what actions you will tolerate and what you will not. Describe in detail the boundaries you want to impose on your interactions with your adult child. Consider Your Values and Needs:

Start by considering your own requirements, principles, and boundaries:Think about what's important to you in terms of your time, personal space, emotional well-being, and other aspects of your life. You can set boundaries that are consistent with your values and that promote your general happiness and wellbeing by using this reflection.

Determine Which Areas Need Boundaries: Determine which areas of your relationship with your adult child require boundaries. Several typical areas include:

Establish your emotional boundaries by deciding how much support you're willing and able to give. Think about how much emotional responsibility you are willing to shoulder and where the line needs to be drawn in order to safeguard your own emotional health.

Limitations of Time and Space: Decide how much time and space you want to spend on yourself. Establish your availability for your adult child, your willingness to spend time with them, and whether you have specific times or days when you need some alone time.

Financial Boundaries: Take into account your financial capabilities and willingness to provide support. Determine what kind of financial support, if any, is affordable and consistent with your values.

Establish your preferences for communication by setting boundaries:Setting rules for frequency, communication channels (such as calls and texts), and respectful communication expectations are all part of this.

Establish Clearly Defined Boundaries: Be clear and precise when defining the boundaries once you've determined which areas call for them. By using "I" statements to express your needs and expectations, make sure your boundaries with your adult child are understood. For instance, "I am here to offer support, but I need you to take responsibility for your own emotions and seek out additional help if you need it" is an example of an emotional boundary.

Example of a Time and Space Boundary: "I value my personal time, and Sundays are necessary for me to unwind and concentrate on myself. On Sundays, I won't be available for visits or long phone calls.

Financial Boundary Example: "I am unable to offer ongoing financial assistance, but I am willing to provide limited financial support for emergencies."

Example of a Communication Boundary: "I like to call you once a week to catch up.

Please let me know if there's an urgent matter so we can arrange a separate conversation.

Consider Obstacles and Exceptions: Recognize that your boundaries may face difficulties or exceptions. Be willing to talk to your adult child about these situations as long as your boundaries are upheld. It's crucial to assess whether each exception fits with your values and abilities on an individual basis.

Consistently enforce your boundaries: It's important to consistently enforce your boundaries. Even if you encounter resistance at first, be adamant about communicating and upholding your boundaries. Consistency promotes the value of your boundaries and aids in the long-term development of healthier dynamics.

Engage in Self-Care: Setting boundaries and taking back control can be emotionally difficult. During this process, give yourself the highest priority. Take part in rejuvenating and health-promoting activities. Ask for assistance from close friends, family, or a therapist who can offer direction and motivation.

Review and modify as necessary: Make sure your boundaries still serve your needs and adhere to your values by periodically reviewing and evaluating them. Be willing to change them if necessary in response to alterations in the situation or shifting dynamics with your adult child.

Be Assertive and Firm: It's important to be assertive and firm when expressing your needs and communicating your boundaries. To avoid ambiguity or misinterpretation, use plain language. Keep in mind that you have the right to set boundaries for your own wellbeing and that they are legitimate.

Active listening is a skill you should develop, along with setting boundaries: Give your adult child a chance to discuss their opinions on boundaries and express their thoughts and feelings. This doesn't imply giving in to pressure to cross boundaries, but it promotes open dialogue and shows that you respect their viewpoint. Keep your non-negotiable boundaries firm, though.

Use "I" Statements: To communicate your needs without coming across as accusatory or judgmental, use "I" statements when setting boundaries. Saying, "You always invade my personal space," for instance, could be replaced with, "I need my personal space to recharge, so I would appreciate it if you could respect that."

Expect Pushback and Be prepared: Your adult child might push back against your attempts to reclaim control and set boundaries. They might be used to a specific dynamic or believe they are entitled to a certain set of privileges. Even if they initially push back, maintain your boundaries with confidence and firmness. Keep in mind that you have the right to set boundaries and put your well being first.

Seek Support: Seeking support from people who have experienced similar things, as well as from therapists or counselors, can be helpful. They can provide direction, suggestions, and validation, which can help you be more determined to establish and uphold boundaries. Online communities or support groups can also foster a sense of camaraderie and understanding.

Establish Repercussions: By establishing repercussions for crossing boundaries, you can emphasize how important it is to respect them. Make the consequences clear and, if necessary, carry them out. Maintaining boundaries and proving that you mean what you say requires consistency.

Practice Self-Compassion: Taking control back from your adult child can result in conflicting feelings, such as guilt or a sense of loss. Self-compassion is a crucial skill to develop during this process. Remind yourself that setting boundaries is a self-care activity that is essential for your general wellbeing. As you travel this journey, be kind to yourself.

Review and Modify Boundaries: It's important to review and modify your boundaries as your relationship with your adult child develops and your circumstances change. Reevaluate your boundaries on a regular basis to see if they are still meeting your needs and if any changes are necessary. Be willing to change, and let your adult child know about these changes.

Do not forget that setting boundaries is a process requiring constant dialogue, introspection, and self-advocacy. You can strengthen your relationship with your adult child and empower yourself by establishing and upholding clear boundaries.

Chapter three

<u>Communicate Openly</u>

Initiate an open and honest conversation with your adult child. Express your concerns, needs, and the importance of establishing healthier dynamics. Clearly communicate your boundaries, making sure your expectations are understood. Encourage a respectful dialogue where both perspectives are heard.

Choose the Right Time and Place: Select an appropriate time and place for a conversation where both you and your adult child can focus without distractions. Ensure there is enough time for a meaningful discussion, and choose a neutral location where both parties feel comfortable.

Approach with Empathy and Respect: Begin the conversation with empathy and respect. Acknowledge that your intention is to improve the relationship and establish healthier dynamics. Frame your discussion around mutual growth and understanding, rather than assigning blame or criticism.

Use "I" Statements: When expressing your thoughts and concerns, use "I" statements to emphasize your personal experience and feelings. This helps to avoid sounding accusatory or confrontational. For example, say, "I feel overwhelmed when I am constantly asked for financial assistance," instead of, "You are always taking advantage of me financially."

Be Specific and Concrete: Clearly articulate your concerns, expectations, and the boundaries you want to establish. Provide specific examples to illustrate your points and make it easier for your adult child to understand your perspective. This specificity helps in avoiding misunderstandings and promotes a more productive dialogue.

Active Listening: Communication is a two-way street. Practice active listening by attentively hearing your adult child's perspective. Give them space to express their thoughts and feelings without interruption. Show genuine interest and empathy towards their point of view. Reflect back what they have shared to ensure understanding.

Validate Their Feelings: Validate your adult child's emotions, even if you may not agree with their actions or behavior. Acknowledge their feelings as valid and important. This validation creates an atmosphere of openness and encourages them to be more receptive to your perspective.

Seek Common Ground: Look for areas of common ground or shared values that can serve as a foundation for rebuilding the relationship. Find points of agreement and understanding to foster a sense of collaboration rather than confrontation. Emphasize the importance of mutual respect and finding a balance that benefits both parties.

Be Solution-Oriented: Instead of dwelling solely on past conflicts or issues, focus on finding solutions and moving forward. Explore strategies and compromises that can help establish healthier dynamics and boundaries. Encourage your adult child to share their thoughts on how the relationship can be improved as well.

Maintain Calm and Composure: It's natural for emotions to run high during such conversations, but strive to maintain a calm and composed demeanor. Take deep breaths, pause when necessary, and avoid getting defensive or aggressive. Responding with calmness and composure sets the tone for a more constructive dialogue.

Establish Follow-up Communication: Conclude the conversation by summarizing the key points discussed and the agreements made. Plan for future communication and check-ins to assess progress and address any concerns. This ongoing communication helps in maintaining accountability and ensures that both parties remain committed to the agreed-upon boundaries.

Practice Patience: Rebuilding a relationship and establishing new dynamics takes time. Patience is key as you navigate through this process. Understand that change may not happen overnight and that setbacks can occur. Be patient with yourself and your adult child as you both adapt to the new boundaries and work towards a healthier relationship.

Use Non-Defensive Language: Avoid becoming defensive or confrontational during the conversation. Stay focused on expressing your thoughts and concerns without attacking or blaming your adult child. Keep the language constructive and solution-oriented to foster a productive dialogue.

Practice Reflective Listening: As your adult child shares their perspective, practice reflective listening by paraphrasing their thoughts and feelings back to them. This shows that you are actively engaged in understanding their point of view and helps to clarify any potential misunderstandings. Reflective listening also demonstrates your commitment to open and respectful communication.

Validate Their Perspective: Show empathy and validation towards your adult child's viewpoint, even if you may not agree with it entirely. Validate their feelings and acknowledge that their perspective has value. This validation helps to create an atmosphere of trust and understanding, allowing for a more fruitful conversation.

Stay Focused on the Issue: During the conversation, it's important to stay focused on the specific issue at hand. Avoid bringing up past conflicts or unrelated matters that may derail the discussion. Keeping the conversation centered on the topic at hand helps maintain clarity and prevents unnecessary tension.

Use "I" Statements for Boundaries: When communicating your boundaries, continue to use "I" statements to assert your needs and expectations. Clearly express how specific behaviors or actions impact you personally, rather than making generalizations or accusations. For example, say, "I feel disrespected when you raise your voice during disagreements," instead of, "You always disrespect me."

Seek Compromise and Collaboration: Emphasize the importance of finding common ground and working together to establish boundaries that are acceptable to both parties. Explore potential compromises that address both your needs and your adult child's concerns. Collaboration fosters a sense of ownership and mutual investment in the relationship.

Maintain Boundaries During the Conversation: As you communicate openly, it's crucial to uphold the boundaries you wish to establish. If your adult child exhibits behavior that crosses those boundaries during the conversation, calmly and assertively reiterate your boundary and remind them of the importance of respecting it. Consistency in maintaining boundaries reinforces their significance and your commitment to self-care.

Address Resistance or Defensiveness: Be prepared for potential resistance or defensiveness from your adult child during the conversation. If they become defensive or try to dismiss your concerns, calmly reiterate the importance of open communication and finding a resolution that benefits both parties. Avoid escalating the situation and strive to keep the conversation focused on understanding and growth.

Practice Emotional Regulation: Throughout the conversation, practice emotional regulation to ensure effective communication. Take deep breaths, remain mindful of your emotions, and pause if necessary to collect your thoughts. Responding with emotional stability helps to maintain a constructive atmosphere and encourages your adult child to engage in open dialogue.

Follow Up with Written Agreement: After the conversation, consider summarizing the key points and agreements reached in a written agreement or email. This serves as a reference point and reminder for both parties. It also helps in ensuring that there is clarity and consensus regarding the boundaries and expectations discussed.

Remember, open communication requires active listening, empathy, and a willingness to understand each other's perspectives. By fostering an environment of open dialogue, you create a foundation for rebuilding trust, mutual respect, and establishing healthier dynamics with your adult child.

Chapter four

<u>Reinforce Consequences</u>

Establish consequences for crossing boundaries or engaging in disrespectful behavior. Communicate these consequences clearly to your adult child, and be prepared to follow through if necessary. Consistency is key in reinforcing boundaries and showing that you mean what you say.

Clearly Define Consequences: Begin by clearly defining the consequences that will be enforced if your adult child crosses established boundaries or engages in disrespectful behavior. Make sure the consequences are specific, fair, and proportional to the situation. This clarity sets clear expectations and reinforces the importance of respecting boundaries.

Communicate Consequences in Advance: Ensure that your adult child is aware of the consequences ahead of time. Clearly communicate the consequences during conversations about boundaries, and reiterate them periodically to reinforce their significance. This allows your adult child to make informed choices and understand the potential outcomes of their actions.

Consistency is Key: Consistency in enforcing consequences is crucial for effective boundary reinforcement. Follow through on the consequences consistently whenever necessary. This consistency sends a message that you are serious about upholding the established boundaries and that actions have real repercussions.

Remain Calm and Objective: When enforcing consequences, it's important to maintain a calm and objective demeanor. Avoid getting overly emotional or engaging in confrontations. Keep the focus on the behavior and its impact rather than attacking the person. By staying calm and objective, you demonstrate that consequences are not driven by anger or retaliation but by the need for respect and healthy boundaries.

Avoid Power Struggles: If your adult child resists or challenges the consequences, avoid getting drawn into power struggles or arguments. Stay firm in your decision while maintaining a respectful and compassionate stance. Reiterate that consequences are in place to protect your well-being and maintain a healthy relationship.

Provide Explanation and Reflection: After enforcing consequences, if appropriate and if your adult child is receptive, provide a clear explanation of why the consequences were necessary. Offer an opportunity for reflection and growth by encouraging them to consider the impact of their behavior on the relationship and the importance of respecting boundaries.

Encourage Accountability and Responsibility: Reinforce the concept of accountability and responsibility by encouraging your adult child to take ownership of their actions. Encourage them to reflect on their behavior, learn from their mistakes, and take steps towards positive change. Emphasize that consequences are an opportunity for growth and personal development.

Offer Supportive Guidance: While consequences are meant to reinforce boundaries, it's important to offer supportive guidance as well. Provide suggestions or resources for your adult child to help them make better choices or seek help if needed. Show that you are willing to support them in their journey towards respectful behavior and personal growth.

Maintain Open Communication: Even when enforcing consequences, maintain open lines of communication with your adult child. Express that while consequences are necessary, your intention is to rebuild a healthy and respectful relationship. Keep the channels of communication open for them to express their thoughts, concerns, or questions, and be willing to listen and engage in dialogue.

Celebrate Positive Changes: Acknowledge and celebrate any positive changes or efforts your adult child makes towards respecting boundaries and improving the relationship. Reinforce their progress with positive reinforcement and encouragement. This helps to build motivation and reinforces the benefits of healthy boundaries and respectful behavior.

Avoid Emotional Manipulation: When enforcing consequences, it's important to avoid engaging in emotional manipulation or guilt-tripping. Stick to the facts and the established consequences without resorting to emotional tactics. This helps maintain fairness and ensures that consequences are based on the behavior itself, rather than on emotional manipulation.

Allow Natural Consequences: Whenever possible, allow natural consequences to occur as a result of your adult child's behavior. Natural consequences are the direct result of their actions and can be powerful learning experiences. Allowing them to experience the natural outcomes of their behavior helps them understand the impact of their actions and can be more effective in promoting change.

Provide an Opportunity for Reflection: After the consequences have been enforced, provide your adult child with an opportunity for reflection. Encourage them to think about their actions, the reasons for the consequences, and the impact it had on the relationship. This self-reflection can foster a deeper understanding and motivate them to make positive changes.

Adjust Consequences if Necessary: If you find that the consequences you initially established are not having the desired effect or if they are too severe, be open to adjusting them. The goal is to find consequences that are effective in promoting positive change and upholding boundaries. Flexibility in adjusting consequences demonstrates a willingness to adapt and find the most suitable approach.

Seek Support: Enforcing consequences can be emotionally challenging, especially when it involves your adult child. Seek support from trusted friends, family members, or professionals, such as therapists or counselors. They can provide guidance, reassurance, and an objective perspective as you navigate through this process.

Remain Firm and Consistent: While it's important to show empathy and provide support, it is equally crucial to remain firm and consistent in reinforcing consequences.

Avoid making exceptions or rescinding consequences due to guilt or pressure. Consistency reinforces the message that boundaries are non-negotiable and that consequences will be enforced when necessary.

Set Boundaries for Yourself: In addition to enforcing consequences for your adult child's behavior, it's important to set boundaries for yourself as well. Establish limits on what you are willing to tolerate and how you will respond if your boundaries are crossed. This self-boundary setting reinforces your commitment to reclaiming power and maintaining a healthy relationship.

Focus on Personal Growth: Emphasize to your adult child that consequences are not solely about punishment but about personal growth and self-improvement. Encourage them to view the consequences as an opportunity for reflection, learning, and making positive changes. Shift the focus from a punitive approach to one that promotes growth, understanding, and healthier dynamics.

Revisit and Reinforce Boundaries Regularly: As the relationship evolves, regularly revisit and reinforce the established boundaries. Have open discussions with your adult child about the progress made, challenges encountered, and any adjustments that may be needed. Consistently reinforcing boundaries helps to maintain a healthy and respectful relationship.

Celebrate Progress: Acknowledge and celebrate any progress your adult child makes in respecting boundaries and improving the relationship. Offer praise, encouragement, and recognition for their efforts. Celebrating progress reinforces the positive changes they are making and strengthens the motivation to continue on the path of growth.

Remember, the purpose of reinforcing consequences is not to punish but to foster growth and establish healthy boundaries. By reinforcing consequences consistently, maintaining empathy, and focusing on personal development, you create an environment that promotes respect, accountability, and positive change within the relationship with your adult child.

Chapter five

<u>Focus on self care</u>

Prioritize self-care to build your emotional strength and resilience. Engage in activities that bring you joy and reduce stress. Seek support from friends, family, or a therapist who can provide guidance and encouragement throughout this process.

Prioritize Self-Awareness: Start by developing a strong sense of self-awareness. Pay attention to your own needs, emotions, and well-being. Recognize when you're feeling overwhelmed, stressed, or drained due to the dynamics with your adult child.

This self-awareness forms the foundation for prioritizing self-care.

Identify Your Self-Care Needs: Reflect on the specific self-care needs that are important to you. Consider activities, practices, or habits that nourish your physical, emotional, and mental well-being. This could include exercise, hobbies, spending time with loved ones, engaging in creative outlets, practicing mindfulness or meditation, or seeking professional support such as therapy.

Establish Boundaries: Set clear boundaries around your personal time, space, and energy. Communicate and enforce these boundaries with your adult child. Let them know when you need alone time or when certain activities are important for your well-being. Respectfully assert your boundaries and prioritize your needs without feeling guilty.

Practice Self-Compassion: Be kind to yourself and practice self-compassion. Understand that it is okay to prioritize your own well-being and establish boundaries for your own mental and emotional health. Release any guilt or feelings of selfishness that may arise. Remind yourself that self-care is essential for your overall happiness and the ability to show up in a healthier way for your adult child.

Develop a Self-Care Routine: Create a regular self-care routine that includes activities or practices that bring you joy, relaxation, and rejuvenation. Dedicate specific time slots in your schedule for self-care activities and make them non-negotiable. Treat self-care as an essential part of your daily or weekly routine, just like any other important commitment.

Seek Support: Reach out to trusted friends, family members, or a therapist for emotional support and guidance. Having a support network can provide a safe space to share your experiences, express your emotions, and gain perspective. Seek professional help if needed to process any challenging emotions or to develop effective coping strategies.

Engage in Stress Reduction Techniques: Incorporate stress reduction techniques into your self-care routine. This could include deep breathing exercises, journaling, practicing mindfulness or meditation, engaging in physical activities, or exploring relaxation techniques such as aromatherapy or listening to calming music. These techniques can help you manage stress and promote emotional well-being.

Set Realistic Expectations: Be mindful of setting realistic expectations for yourself.

Understand that you cannot control or change your adult child's behavior entirely. Focus on what is within your control—your own well-being, boundaries, and responses. Let go of the need to fix everything and instead shift your energy towards taking care of yourself.

Create a Supportive Environment: Surround yourself with a supportive and understanding environment. Spend time with people who uplift and encourage you. Engage in activities and environments that foster positivity and nourish your well-being. Consider joining support groups or online communities where you can connect with others who are navigating similar experiences.

Regularly Assess and Adjust: Regularly assess your self-care routine and adjust as needed. Check in with yourself to see if the activities and practices you engage in are truly nurturing your well-being. Be open to trying new things and exploring different self-care strategies that resonate with you. Self-care is a dynamic process that evolves as your needs change.

Practice Mindfulness: Incorporate mindfulness into your self-care routine. Engage in activities that allow you to be fully present in the moment, such as practicing meditation, going for mindful walks in nature, or engaging in mindful eating. Mindfulness helps to cultivate awareness, reduce stress, and promote overall well-being.

Establish Healthy Boundaries with Others: In addition to setting boundaries with your adult child, it's important to establish healthy boundaries with other people in your life. This includes friends, family members, and even your own support network. Ensure that your relationships are based on mutual respect, understanding, and reciprocity. Set boundaries to protect your time, energy, and emotional well-being.

Nurture Healthy Habits: Focus on nurturing healthy habits that support your physical and mental well-being. This includes getting regular exercise, prioritizing nutritious meals, getting enough sleep, and engaging in activities that promote relaxation and stress reduction. Taking care of your physical health provides a strong foundation for overall well-being.

Engage in Creative Outlets: Explore creative outlets as a form of self-expression and self-care. Engaging in activities such as painting, writing, playing music, or pursuing any other creative interests can be therapeutic and allow for emotional release.

Creativity can also serve as a source of joy, fulfillment, and personal growth.

Learn to Say No: Practice the art of saying no when necessary. Be selective with your commitments and prioritize activities that align with your values and well-being. Saying no to excessive demands or responsibilities that deplete your energy allows you to create space for self-care and focus on what truly matters to you.

Unplug and Disconnect: Dedicate regular periods of time to unplug from technology and disconnect from the constant stream of notifications and information. Engage in activities that foster quiet introspection, such as reading a book, practicing meditation, or spending time in nature. Disconnecting helps to reduce mental clutter and create space for rejuvenation.

Embrace Self-Reflection: Engage in self-reflection to gain deeper insights into your own needs, desires, and personal growth. Set aside time for journaling or introspection to explore your thoughts, feelings, and experiences. Self-reflection allows you to gain clarity, identify patterns, and make intentional choices that align with your well-being.

Celebrate Achievements: Take time to acknowledge and celebrate your achievements, big or small. Recognize your progress in reclaiming power and establishing healthy boundaries with your adult child. Celebrating achievements reinforces a positive mindset and boosts self-confidence, fostering a sense of accomplishment and motivation to continue prioritizing self-care.

Practice Self-Compassion: Be gentle and compassionate with yourself throughout the journey of reclaiming power. Acknowledge that it is a process that may involve ups and downs. Offer yourself understanding, forgiveness, and kindness when facing challenges or setbacks. Practice self-compassion as a way to nurture self-care and cultivate resilience.

Regularly Reconnect with Joy: Engage in activities that bring you joy and ignite a sense of passion and fulfillment. This could include hobbies, spending time with loved ones, pursuing interests, or engaging in activities that make you laugh and feel alive. Reconnecting with joy fuels your spirit, renews your energy, and enhances your overall well-being.

Remember, focusing on self-care is not selfish but essential for your own well-being and the ability to navigate the challenges of reclaiming power from your adult child. By prioritizing self-care, you cultivate resilience, inner strength, and a healthier mindset that will support you in creating a more balanced and harmonious relationship.

Chapter six

<u>Seek professional help if needed</u>

If the situation remains challenging or escalates, consider seeking professional help from a family therapist or counselor. They can offer insights, guidance, and mediation to help you and your adult child navigate through difficult issues and establish healthier patterns of interaction.

Recognize the Need for Professional Help: Acknowledge that seeking professional help can be beneficial when navigating complex family dynamics and reclaiming power from your adult child. It shows a proactive commitment to your own well-being and the health of your relationship.

Research Different Professionals: Start by researching professionals who specialize in areas such as family therapy, relationship counseling, or parental guidance. Look for those who have experience working with adult children and can provide the support you need. Consider factors like their qualifications, expertise, and the therapeutic approaches they use.

Seek Recommendations: Ask for recommendations from trusted sources, such as your primary care physician, friends, or family members who may have sought similar support. Their insights can help you narrow down your options and find professionals who are highly regarded and trustworthy.

Consider Accessibility and Compatibility: Take into account practical considerations, such as the location, availability, and affordability of professionals you're considering. Additionally, consider their compatibility with your communication style, values, and approach to therapy. It's important to feel comfortable and connected with the professional you choose.

Initial Consultation: Schedule an initial consultation with the professional you're interested in working with. This meeting allows you to gauge their expertise, their understanding of your situation, and their suitability for your needs. Prepare a list of questions or concerns to discuss during this consultation.

Be Open and Honest: During the initial consultation and subsequent sessions, be open and honest about your situation, goals, and concerns. Provide relevant details about your relationship with your adult child and the power dynamics you're seeking to address. Clear communication ensures that the professional has a comprehensive understanding of your needs.

Assess Their Approach: Inquire about the professional's therapeutic approach and how they typically work with clients facing similar challenges. Discuss their views on boundaries, communication, and empowerment. Ensure that their approach aligns with your values and goals for reclaiming power in the relationship.

Collaborative Relationship: Seek a professional who emphasizes a collaborative and empowering therapeutic relationship. It's important to find someone who encourages your active involvement, values your input, and works with you to develop strategies and goals. A collaborative approach fosters a sense of ownership and personal growth.

Regular Communication: Once you've chosen a professional, establish a schedule and frequency of sessions that work for you. Commit to regular communication and attend sessions consistently. Consistency enhances the effectiveness of therapy and provides a supportive structure as you navigate the process of reclaiming power.

Set Realistic Expectations: Understand that change takes time and effort. Set realistic expectations for the therapeutic process and the progress you hope to make. Recognize that setbacks and challenges may arise along the way, but with perseverance, you can work through them and continue moving forward.

Active Participation: Actively participate in the therapeutic process. Engage in discussions, complete any suggested exercises or homework, and reflect on the insights gained. Be open to exploring new perspectives and implementing suggested strategies. Your active participation enhances the effectiveness of therapy.

Evaluate Progress: Periodically evaluate your progress and the effectiveness of the professional help you're receiving. Assess whether the therapeutic approach is aligning with your goals and if you're experiencing positive changes in your relationship with your adult child. If needed, discuss any concerns or adjustments with the professional.

Explore Different Modalities: There are various therapeutic modalities that professionals may specialize in, such as cognitive-behavioral therapy (CBT), family systems therapy, psychodynamic therapy, or solution-focused therapy. Research and explore these different modalities to understand which approach may resonate with you and your specific needs.

Address Emotional Impact: Recognize that the process of reclaiming power from your adult child can evoke a range of emotions. A skilled professional can help you navigate and process these emotions in a safe and supportive environment. They can provide guidance on managing feelings of guilt, anger, sadness, or frustration that may arise during this journey.

Develop Coping Strategies: Work with the professional to develop effective coping strategies that can help you manage stress, anxiety, or any challenges that arise as you reclaim power. These strategies may include relaxation techniques, mindfulness exercises, communication skills, or emotional regulation tools. Having coping strategies in place can enhance your resilience and well-being.

Explore Communication Techniques: Professionals can help you develop effective communication techniques to assert boundaries, express your needs, and navigate difficult conversations with your adult child. They can provide guidance on active listening, assertive communication, and conflict resolution skills that promote healthier dialogue and foster understanding.

Foster a Supportive Therapeutic Relationship: Building a strong therapeutic relationship with your professional is essential for a successful journey of reclaiming power. Ensure that you feel heard, validated, and supported during your sessions. Trust and rapport between you and the professional can create a safe space for exploration, growth, and healing.

Track Progress and Celebrate Achievements: Keep track of your progress throughout your therapeutic journey. Reflect on the positive changes, insights gained, and milestones achieved along the way. Celebrate your achievements, no matter how small, as they signify your growth and resilience in reclaiming power from your adult child.

Engage in Homework or Assignments: Professionals may provide homework assignments or activities to reinforce what you discuss during sessions. Embrace these assignments as opportunities for self-reflection, practice, and integration of new skills. Completing these tasks can deepen your understanding and enhance the effectiveness of therapy.

Communicate Any Concerns: If at any point during therapy you have concerns or doubts about the approach, progress, or dynamics with the professional, openly communicate them. Honest communication fosters a collaborative relationship and allows for adjustments, if necessary, to ensure the therapy aligns with your needs.

Involve Your Adult Child, if Appropriate: Depending on the circumstances, it may be helpful to involve your adult child in therapy sessions. With the guidance of your professional, you can engage in family therapy or invite your adult child to join a session to facilitate open communication, understanding, and reconciliation. This can promote a shared commitment to growth and healing.

Embrace Personal Growth: Embrace the personal growth that occurs throughout the therapeutic process. Recognize that this journey is not solely about reclaiming power from your adult child but also about your own self-discovery, healing, and transformation. Embrace the opportunity to cultivate self-awareness, resilience, and healthier relationship dynamics.

Be Patient with the Process: Therapy is a process that takes time, and progress may occur at different rates. Be patient and compassionate with yourself as you navigate the complexities of reclaiming power. Remember that healing and change require patience, commitment, and an understanding that progress may come in small steps rather than immediate transformations.

Continually Reevaluate Your Needs: As you progress through therapy, regularly reevaluate your needs and goals. Discuss any shifts or changes in your circumstances, challenges that arise, or new insights gained with your professional. This allows for adjustments to be made in the therapeutic approach to better address your evolving needs.

Maintain Boundaries with the Professional: While therapy involves a close professional relationship, it's important to maintain appropriate boundaries. Remember that the professional's role is to guide and support you, and their personal involvement in your life should be limited to the therapeutic context. Maintain professional boundaries to ensure a healthy therapeutic dynamic.

Utilize Therapy as a Supportive Resource: Even after reaching your goals or making significant progress, consider therapy as a supportive resource that you can return to if needed. Life circumstances may change, and having a trusted professional to turn to during challenging times can provide ongoing support and guidance.

Remember, seeking professional help is a valuable step towards reclaiming power and establishing healthier dynamics in your relationship with your adult child. A skilled professional can provide guidance, support, and tools to navigate the complexities of family dynamics and empower you in this journey.